Mediterranean Diet Cookbook

70 Top Mediterranean Diet Recipes & Meal Plan

JOHN JAMES

Table of content

The term Mediterranean diet refers to a selected combination of foods made in antioxidants, minerals, and vitamins along with an ideal balance of fatty acids. However, it's going to not be classified joined of the standard meal plans followed to attain targeted health outcomes, particularly weight loss. In fact, Mediterranean diet (MD) isn't near to ingestion food as you cannot eat your manner for weight loss or for higher health. MD is really a harmony of diet and modus vivendi which ends in a very healthy life balance ever elusive in much all regions of the planet except Ella's, Crete, European country and Spain. The latter regions are typically geographically known because the Mediterranean basin.

The Mediterranean diet isn't just a furor because it has been in observe since past times within the region. Whereas furor diets vanish to oblivion in only a brief span of your time, MD persisted through the years. Its vaunted effectuality for an extended list of health advantages evolved from tradition and viva-voce to on trial claims and conjectures, till research project documented the link between typical food consumed by a selected population on one hand and their longevity and low prevalence of chronic and coronary diseases on the opposite hand. MD is that the collection of food enclosed within the diet, however food is eaten, and the way numerous fascinating practices are synergized to form a potent life balance for healthy living. Therefore, MD could also be a lot of suitably observed because the Mediterranean healthy modus vivendi.
As readers would have noticed, the region wherever the MD originated includes of many teams of culturally completely different individuals. However, despite marked changes in their ancient diets and luxury foods, the individuals during this region are awake to the importance of enjoying their meal and whenever potential, they get pleasure from a hearty noon meal with the entire family.

Chapter one presents the twelve basic guiding principles of the Mediterranean diet. The advantages of adopting the Mediterranean diet for one's health are explained in Chapter two. Chapter three introduces the reader to a special Two-Week Weight Loss set up supported the principles of this heart-friendly diet. Meanwhile, Chapter four offers suggestions concerning the manner way to stock the house buttery and therefore the refrigerator of goodies for getting ready meals the Mediterranean way. Chapter five presents feeding out ideas for people or families reliably signed to the Mediterranean diet.
The maintenance plan for the two-week weight loss initiative is unclothed in Chapter six. basic cognitive process that healthy youngsters are the happiest children, the seventh chapter of the book is devoted to foods within the Mediterranean diet that are nice for youths. Chapter eight carries the highlight of this eBook, luxurious recipes of dishes within the ancient tailor-fitted for the weight-loss set up victimization the low- carbs approach.

The Mediterranean diet organic phenomenon is additionally shown during this chapter. The recipes options dishes categorized in terms of the following: fish, dessert, legumes, meat, alimentary paste / rice / bread, poultry, salad, snack, soup, and vegetables. Bonus chapters on the information for Mediterranean change of state caps your healthy scan.

Enjoy the food and keep healthy the Mediterranean way

Consume Lots of Fruits

There isn't any limit in regards to the selection of fruits to include inside the MD. However, since culmination include nutrients and nutrients in special quantities, it is always higher to go along with darkish-colored end result, which nutritionists claim to supply an more-normal dietary punch. Dark-colored fruits particularly the darkish crimson and orange ones, and even veggies provide anti-oxidants and phyto- nutrients. Variety is likewise an vital aspect in choosing fruits for the MD.

The following fruits are usually grown within the Mediterranean: figs, grapes, lemons, mandarin oranges, olives, persimmons, and pomegranates. Other important culmination inside the MD are blackberries, blueberries, cranberries, plums, red grapes, and crimson raspberries. MD experts also recommend succulent or those containing lots of fiber and water, such as: apples, oranges, peaches, and watermelons. The idea behind more water and fiber in the diet is to help weight watchers experience glad longer and to aid in the digestive process.

Whereas there is no limit to the choice of fruits which may be included in the weight loss plan, servings will ought to be controlled. Moreover, there ought to be extra veggies than end result in the weight loss plan, for two foremost reasons: first, culmination have extra calories than vegetables; and second, end result do not have much range of nutrients than veggies. One and a half of servings of end result an afternoon is typical in MD. The serving size of most end result except banana is one cup. One 8- to 9- inch banana is one serving. Fruit juices or canned end result can be substituted for raw culmination at one cup in line with serving, while one serving of dried culmination is equal to one-1/2 cup

Consume Lots of Vegetables

All vegetables can be included in the MD, however people need to attempt to restrict their intake of corn and white potatoes because of their high starch content, which in turn contribute to extra calories. The following greens are commonly grown inside the Mediterranean: artichokes, asparagus, broccoli, broccoli rabe, cabbage, eggplant, green beans, garlic, onions, and tomatoes. Dark-colored vegetables along with beets, carrots, purple peppers, and sweet potatoes are super sources of anti-oxidants and phyto-nutrients. Likewise, eat masses of inexperienced, leafy veggies aside from broccoli due to the fact these also are powerhouses of nutrients: bok choy, cauliflower, collards, kale, lettuce, mustard, romaine, spinach, summer time and wintry weather squash, turnip vegetables and zucchini.

Broccoli rabe is also referred to as broccoli raab or rapini. Broccoli rabe is also called broccoli raab or rapini.

Collard is also referred to as non-heading cabbage or tree-cabbage Collard is also called non-heading cabbage or tree-cabbage

Adults need to consume at the least cups of veggies in the MD. Vegetables can be eaten raw,
cooked or using them as elements to different dishes. For those who would love to strive the MD howev;er are hesitating due to the fact they don't want to eat loads of vegetables might be glad to recognise that vegetable serving sizes do now not need to be large. The following common vegetable consumption requirements can also serve as your manual in getting ready food the Mediterranean way. The good information is, it conforms to the dietary pointers of health and nutrition authorities:

At least 1 ½ cups of orange-colored greens in keeping with week At least 2 cups according to week of darkish inexperienced greens

At least 5 ½ cups in line with week of other vegetables

For the ones trying the MD for healthy eating, at least 2 ½ cups in keeping with week of starchy veggies, however the ones doing the MD for weight loss must refrain from or limit intake of starch-rich veggies to a maximum of one cup in a week.

Consume Legumes

Legumes are complete within the macronutrients carbohydrates, proteins, and fats and oils, whereas end result and vegetables do now not have fat and oils. Legumes are also wealthy in vitamins B1, B3, B6, and B9 and in minerals inclusive of calcium, magnesium, and molybdenum. The following legumes are usually grown within the Mediterranean: chickpeas, lentils, and peas. However, legumes for inclusion within the MD are infinite and may also encompass black beans, black-eyed peas, fantastic northern beans, kidney beans, and cut up beans.

For the ones who aren't fond of consuming legumes, you can choose simply and add those in your soups and stews. Legumes add a variety of taste in food, gives your fiber needs, and have very little fat. At least 2½ cups of legumes per week are required inside the MD.

Include Nuts and Seeds for your Diet

Nuts and seeds are a staple in Mediterranean cuisine, both as the principle element in a snack recipe or to add fantastic flavor to food. The following nuts typically grown in the Mediterranean are: almonds, hazelnuts, pine nuts, and walnuts. Other healthy nuts and seeds which are indispensable in the MD are: Brazil nuts, cashew nuts, chia seeds, flaxseeds or linseeds, macadamia nuts, peanuts (even though peanuts are certainly legumes), pecan nuts, pistachio nuts, pumpkin seeds, sesame seeds, and sunflower seeds. Quinoa (absolutely now not a true cereal but a pseudocereal) may be taken into consideration a seed.

With all the remarkable advantages which may be derived from nuts and seeds especially healthy fat, those food items also incorporate calories. Those who are looking their weight or are following the MD weight-reduction plan for weight loss need to control their intake of nuts and seeds.

Here are approximate numbers of a few nuts that normally include an ounce - the everyday serving size of nuts:

Almonds: 20 to 25

Brazil nuts: 6 to 8

Cashew nuts: 16 to 18

Hazel nuts: 10 to 12

Peanuts: 28

Pecan nuts: 15 halves Pine nuts: 50 to 157

Pistachios: forty five to 47

Walnuts: 14 halves

A caveat approximately nuts: Brazil nuts, cashew nuts and peanuts have higher content material of unhealthy fats. The high-quality nuts are almonds and walnuts because of their Omega 3 content and their splendid taste. Nuts are satisfactory when they're raw, but if you virtually needed to cook them then go for toasted nuts. Also ensure that they may be unsalted and uncoated, and with no brought sugar and fat. Also, the claims about chia seeds have not but been scientifically proven, so they should be ate up in mild servings of one ounce at the most

Eat entire grains, in particular whole grain bread Technically, the term whole grain refers back to the grain or method grain products wherein the caryopsis such as the anatomical components bran, germ and endosperm are intact whether they're ground, cracked, or flaked. Whole grains are necessary to the MD as they contain excessive quantities of fiber and impart natural goodness to food. Among the entire grain produce commonplace within the Mediterranean region are: barley, corn, rice, and wheat. If you like bread, select dense, heavy chewy breads baked from while wheat, barley, and oats. If you love pasta, pick out complete grain pasta products from the grocery store.

There are many motives for deciding on entire grain foods no longer simplest for his or her health blessings but additionally for that feeling of fullness you want for your each day routines. MD experts additionally endorse steel-cut, entire-grain oatmeal and multi-grain hot cereals. The good information with MD is that it lets in humans a wide preference of whole grains. Even people who love rice can enjoy ingesting rice so long as they chose brown rice. Couscous and polenta are also amazing entire grain choices. Whole grains are an critical a part of the Mediterranean diet.

Whole grains are an fundamental a part of the Mediterranean weight-reduction plan.

Use Olive Oil in Cooking and in Salads

Olive oil is the main fat supply used within the MD. Thus, the consumption of olive oil in Mediterranean international locations is excessive even of other less expensive oils are becoming famous. With the cutting-edge interest in MD, even non-Mediterranean international locations together with Germany, Japan, UK and US have increasing consumption of olive oil. Olive oil defines the distinctive taste of the MD and is therefore of precise significance within the average context of the MD.

Olive oil now not most effective increases the palatability of foods however also improves the feel and complements the taste. In Greece, the very famous lathera dish consists of veggies cooked in an olive oil-based totally sauce, tomatoes, and garlic. Leading government at the MD believes that without the use of olive oil within the instruction of Mediterranean dishes, it might be practically impossible for humans in Greece and inside the surrounding international locations inside the area to consume high quantities of greens and legumes.

Olive oil is used inside the Mediterranean weight-reduction plan no longer most effective for cooking however additionally for the following functions among others:

Raw olive oil is used in aiolli and other dips; Vegetable marinades;

Flavoring for soups and stews by using long, slow cooking, specially in pistou; For batter, dough, and numerous pastries;

Bread with oil, which is taken into consideration as elemental Mediterranean cuisine, which includes the Catalan dish pa amb oli.

Mediterranean people very not often use butter in their cuisine and they do no longer omit it because olive oil has its simple appeal for his or her dishes. In activities in which olive oil does no longer suit a particular recipe, canola oil is used instead. Extra virgin olive oil, mainly the lighter model is the nice preference for salad dressings, for use in meals eaten raw, and in baking. However, for cooking, everyday extra virgin oil to be had in the supermarket is just fine. One should no longer hesitate to put together foods the Mediterranean way due to the price of olive oil because it will replace butter and margarine. The small fee delivered in the use of olive is nothing as compared to its health advantages.

Include Moderate Amounts of Low Fat Dairy or If Possible, Non-Fat Dairy

In the Mediterranean, goat and sheep milk are extra desired than cow's milk. However, as long as you select low-fat or non-fat milk, it's miles good sufficient for inclusion within the MD. Rather than the standard Western cheese, yogurt is a very crucial constituent of the MD, collectively with some difficult and soft forms of cheese. Greek yogurt has a rich silky texture and is widely available in many supermarkets within the US. It is a better desire because it has two times the protein content of regular commercial yogurt however expenses the same as the name-brand ordinary yogurt.

There is even fat-unfastened Greek yogurt for weight-watchers which is already available within the US. Even Starbucks has jumped into the Greek yogurt bandwagon and is teaming up with a Greek yogurt manufacturer. By subsequent year, Americans established with the healthful Mediterranean weight loss program can buy ready- to-consume Greek yogurt parfaits from the multi-chain international espresso store. Meanwhile, the MD isn't always acknowledged for its heavy use of cheese. Rather, cheese is used extra as a flavoring to decorate the taste of food, however now not necessarily to crush it. Cheese is also utilized in MD in combination with dessert. If you want cheese, make certain that it is also the low-fats variety and consume dairy products in moderation

Eat Fish and Shellfish

Influenced by way of geography, the Mediterranean weight loss program includes seafood as one in every of its crucial components. Moreover, the selection of fish inside the traditional eating regimen is largely responsible for the coronary heart-healthy popularity of the MD weight loss program. Fish like cod, haddock, mackerel, red mullet, salmon, and sardines, which can be cold-water fish varieties, are rich in Omega 3 and different unsaturated fats. Squid and octopus also are staple seafood inside the MD. Consuming fish with high Omega three rather than animal meats guarantees that the body's arteries are not clogged and are protected from coronary diseases.

Other fish now not essential from the Mediterranean which might be rich in Omega 3 and unsaturated fats are Albacore tuna, anchovies, Arctic char or iwana, Atlantic mackerel, sablefish or black cod, Pacific halibut, rainbow trout, shad, smelt, and wild salmon. Shellfish are also welcome in the MD. Among the healthiest are clams, crab, lobster, mussels, oysters, scallops, and shrimps.

Include the Right (Healthy) Fats to your Diet

Not all fat are terrible for one's fitness. In fact, most those who study and/or examine about the MD see that Mediterranean human beings do now not always devour a low-fats food regimen. However, research proof along with the findings of the look at conducted with the aid of the Keys husband-and-wife crew showed that these people have healthy coronary heart conditions. The explanation for this phenomenon lies within the intake of healthier types of fats together with monounsaturated fats and polyunsaturated omega 3 fatty acids. These are the right forms of fat that ought to be included in the food regimen.

Make Physical Activity Part of your Daily Routine

A appropriate dose of every day physical hobby is part of the Mediterranean lifestyle. The MD will not be as effective as it's miles for folks who do no longer like to take pleasure in physical activity in workout on a everyday basis. The rural oldsters from the Mediterranean region do no longer care about doing aerobics or cardio exercises. However, they have masses of day by day physical interest through the work they interact in, travelling where they had to cross on foot, and having fun. Modern residing in any part of the world may not always allow human beings to do what the Mediterranean oldsters do, but they can benefit from the MD through running out, doing aerobic exercises, and engaging in electricity schooling exercises

Drink Wine in Moderate Amounts

Red wine is recommended, however not a "must" in the Mediterranean diet. It provides protection to the heart from the anti-oxidants from flavonoids within the skin of the grapes. Flavonoids decrease the chance of heart disease as it lowers horrific cholesterol, increases appropriate cholesterol, and reduces blood clotting inside the arteries. Studies are now underway to verify another health enjoy the flavonoid known as resveratrol, also determined in purple wine. It is alleged that resveratrol inhibits tumor development in sure cancers.

In location of red wine for individuals who do now not drink alcoholic drinks, grape juice made from Concord grapes paintings just as fine. Likewise, ingesting purple grapes also gives the same benefits for a wholesome heart. As a count number of precaution, however, the recommended every day intake together with the MD is four ounces each day for girls and two 4-ounce intakes for men. Like any other food, anything fed on in extra influences the health negatively. Excessive consuming even of purple wine will bring about hypertension, cardiovascular conditions, and extra calories.

Red wine inside the MD is recommended most effective for people who are in desirable health. Never consume alcohol if you have been prescribed a day by day dose of aspirin for a medical situation. If you've got any of the following conditions, you aren't to drink any alcoholic liquids as doing so will cause your situation to worsen:

Congestive heart failure; High triglycerides level Hypertension (excessive blood pressure); Liver disease; and/or Pancreatitis.

Eat Very Small Servings of Red Meat Occasionally

In the Mediterranean weight-reduction plan, red meat is ate up rarely, as in most effective a couple of times a week. However,

for clarity, the servings need to be limited. If you need to have red meat twice a week, make certain you consume no greater than a complete of 12 oz. for the week. Lean cuts need to be ate up, which shows that the fat portion wishes to be trimmed out. If you use red meat as element to soup or pasta, this need to remember as a part of the 12 ounces limit in step with week.

People may feel that they are significantly confined in their pork consumption. They are right. However, the limit is essential because beef is a main contributing element to cancer, heart ailment, and stroke. After all, you do no longer embark on a Mediterranean eating regimen just to savour the delectable cuisine of the region. You are doing it for your fitness.

In the groundbreaking Seven Countries Study of the Nineteen Fifties conducted via Ancel and Margaret Keys, outcomes showed the association among the form of food human beings eat on one hand, and lifestyles expectancy and the superiority of chronic and coronary sicknesses on the alternative hand. The have a look at turned into conducted in the Mediterranean region. The findings tested that consumption of food significantly low in fat leads to higher lifestyles expectancy and very low incidence of chronic diseases, especially persistent heart ailment. From thereon, interest become targeted at the beneficial results of the Mediterranean food regimen. This marked the foundation of the idea of the Mediterranean diet (MD).

Based at the dialogue in Chapter 1, readers will not really associate MD with a vegetarian or vegan eating regimen. With fish, meat, and dairy components, the MD is delightfully flavorful and abounds in hedonistic qualities. Yet, the diets were frugal and do now not have excessive calories. Adding up to the moderate calorie intake is regular physical interest, although now not exactly the concept of physical pastime popular within the gyms of Western countries, but extensive sufficient to result in lower quotes of obesity within the Mediterranean region. Thus, the wholesome Mediterranean way of life become idea to be some thing accurate to emulate.

Further research later buttressed the Keys' findings and a roster of fitness benefits were compiled. In no time, a new and effective regimen for health and longevity was born. This bankruptcy summarizes the useful results of the Mediterranean eating regimen. Results of 3 recent studies showed that:

From a examine published in the British Medical Journal in the yr 2008, following the conventional MD led to a 9◆creased in deaths from coronary artery disease.

In 2011, a systematic assessment published in the Journal of the American College of Cardiology related to 535,000 cases discovered that traditional MD is correlated with lower blood pressure, and decrease ranges blood glucose and triglycerides.

In early 2013, a look at among 7,447 instances of high danger of cardiovascular situations showed no sizable difference among 3 companies within the discount of risk for coronary heart attack, stroke, and heart disorder. Two organizations both accompanied the conventional MD but one group become supplemented with olive, even as the alternative turned into complement with nuts. The third institution accompanied a low-fats weight loss plan.

As compiled with the aid of Denver physician Eric Zacharias in 2012, MD is effective within the prevention of weight problems and in weight loss. From the same compilation, Dr. Zacharias also mentioned that the MD is associated with reduced universal mortality charge and reduced danger for some of medical conditions including:

Allergic rhinitis Alzheimer's disease Arthritis

Asthma Atopy Cancer

Cardiovascular illnesses Dementia

Depression

Macular degeneration (age-related) Metabolic syndrome

Parkinson's disease

Rheumatoid arthritis Type 2 diabetes

Other fitness advantages of the MD with appreciate to better first-rate of existence include: Healthy aging

Healthy vision Improved reminiscence Strong bones and enamel Stronger immune system

Chapter three Mediterranean Diet: Two Weeks Weight Loss Plan

Week 1 Weight Loss Plan Day 1: Sunday

Breakfast

Grape Juice

Chickpea and Barley Glee Fruit in season or pear

Morning Snack
Pumpkin seeds

Lunch

Lamb Loin Chops
Fruit in season or orange Red wine or cranberry juice

Afternoon Snack
Fruity Smoothie No. 1

Dinner

Baked Salmon with Honey-Balsamic Glaze Fruit in season
Red wine or apple juice (if you had pink wine for lunch have apple juice or another MD
fruit guidelines for dinner)

Day 2: Monday Breakfast
Lemon Juice
Apple-Walnut Delight
Fruit in season or persimmon Morning Snack
Quinoa

Lunch

Salmon-Asparagus Omelet (Frittata) Fruit in season or plums
Red wine or orange juice

Afternoon Snack
Fruity Smoothie No. 2

Dinner

Broiled halibut
Fruit in season or peaches
Red wine or orange juice (if you had crimson wine for lunch have orange juice or some
other MD fruit recommendations for dinner)

Day three: Tuesday Breakfast
Non-fats goat's milk Breakfast Rush Fruit in season
Morning Snack

Lunch

Flaxseeds

Sesame Tuna Temptation Fruit in season
Four seasons herbal juice (homemade, juice four of your favorite culmination and drink)

Afternoon Snack
Fruity Smoothie No. 3

Dinner

Grilled Shrimp Fruit in season Red wine punch

Day 4: Wednesday Breakfast
Breakfast Rush Fruit in season
Morning Snack
Snack Pack (half of the serving for breakfast, see recipe on Chapter eight for Breakfast
Rush.)

Lunch

Sesame Tuna Temptation Fruit in season Pineapple juice

Afternoon Snack
Frutti Smoothie No. 4

Dinner

Steamed Oysters Fruit in season Fruit punch

Day 5: Thursday Breakfast
Fruit Salad Mediterranean Style Brown Rice and Stuffed Chicken Carrot Soup
Morning Snack
Chia seeds

Lunch

Lentil soup Fruit in season
Chili Chicken and Beans

Afternoon Snack
Savory Mixed Nuts

Dinner

Lime Chicken Fruit in season
Celery and fennel soup

Day 6: Friday

Breakfast

Hot Lemon and Honey Walnut Baklava
Fruit in season

Morning Snack
Fruity Smoothie 5

Lunch

Fish Stew in Saffron and White Beans Fruit in season
Red wine

Afternoon Snack
Walnut Baklava (half of serving)

Dinner

Grouper in Tomato-Olive Sauce Eggplant and Tomato Pesto Turkey Soup

Day 7: Saturday Breakfast
Non-fat milk
Mixed Vegetable Omelet Fruit in season
Morning Snack
Mixed nuts and seeds (half cup)

Lunch

Salmon and Cashew Fruit in season Tomato soup

Afternoon Snack
Fruity Smoothie 3

Dinner

Fennel, White Beans and Seared Salmon Frutti Smoothie No. 6
Green soup

Week 2 Weight Loss Plan Day 1: Sunday
Breakfast
Fruity Smoothie No. 6 Bean and sausage soup Poached fish
Morning Snack
Pistachios and pecan nuts

Lunch

Fish curry and veggies Fruit in season Minestrone soup

Afternoon Snack
Fruity Smoothie No. 7

Dinner

Zucchini Gratin Fruit in season
Fish and Seafood Primavera

Day 2: Monday Breakfast
Rice Pudding
Pepper and Red Snapper Fruit in season
Morning Snack
Almonds or walnuts

Lunch

Ground Round Special Ale Turk Lettuce and cucumber salad
Red wine or orange juice

Afternoon Snack
Banana

Dinner
Tuna Casserole
Fruit in season or peaches Pumpkin and sweet potato soup

Day three: Tuesday Breakfast
Whole grain oats (rolled) Non-fats or skim milk Fruit in season
Morning Snack
A little Feta cheese and whole grain bread

Lunch
Roasted Vegetable Chowder Fruit Salad Mediterranean-Style Mediterranean Tuna

Afternoon Snack
Apples and grapes

Dinner
Grilled Mediterranean Seafood with S-dip Fruit in season
Potato Leek Soup

Day 4: Wednesday Breakfast
Mediterranean Toast Fruity Smoothie No. eight Apple juice
Morning Snack
Quinoa salad

Lunch
Chicken Chili Fruit in season Pea soup

Afternoon Snack
Cucumber in natural sweetened vinegar

Dinner
Pasta and Sardines Fruity Smoothie No. nine Cabbage soup
Red wine

Day 5: Thursday Breakfast
Greek salad Grape juice Grilled seafood
Morning Snack
Soy milk

Lunch
Marinated mushroom Fruit in season or orange
Mediterranean salmon or tuna

Afternoon Snack
Fruity Smoothie No. 9

Dinner
Stuffed Tomatoes Shrimp and pasta Red wine

Day 6: Friday Breakfast
Sugar-free gelato
Mediterranean low-cholesterol pizza Fruit in season
Morning Snack
Peaches

Lunch
Greek seafood burger Fruit in season Orange juice

Afternoon Snack
fruity Smoothie No. 10
Dinner
Stuffed Pepper Roast

Fruit in season
Bourbon-glazed tuna or salmon Kale and chook soup

Day 7: Saturday Breakfast
Pumpkin and corn muffin Fruit in season
Walnut milk Morning Snack
Quinoa mild salad

Lunch

Mediterranean seafood stew Fruit in season
Pasta and shrimps

Afternoon Snack
Pumpkin and corn muffin

Dinner
Grilled Vegetable salad Fruit in season Poached shellfish
Red wine punch
Chapter four How to Stock Pantry and Fridge
The Mediterranean food plan emphasizes the usage of fresh food items instead of
processed (i.E., canned) merchandise if this may be helped. However, there are a few
staples which want to be saved at hand within the refrigerator or in the pantry. Many
convenience meals and snacks for the food plan needed to be stored cold. Fresh produce
may be kept in a fridge.
Stuff for the Refrigerator and Freezer
Following are the basic items which individuals or families following the Mediterranean
diet regimen have to continually have ready inside the fridge:
Bread and rolls; Carton of eggs;

Fresh vegetables, inclusive of carrots, celery, and lettuce; Honey or maple syrup;
Cheese (sourced from goat or sheep); Greek yogurt, both normal and low-fat; 1-percent
milk or cottage cheese;
Nuts
Natural nut butters consisting of peanuts and almond butter
Condiments inclusive of Cayenne or Tabasco sauce, mustard sauce, Worcestershire
sauce, salsas, and mayonnaise.
Weekly food supplies from the supermarket such as fish, chicken, and meat need to
usually be saved within the freezer. Frozen products together with frozen berries, frozen
vegetables, and frozen shrimps should additionally be stored inside the freezer right after
shopping.
Meanwhile, minced garlic and minced ginger must be stored within the refrigerator. For
bigger amounts of minced garlic, the freezer affords a higher garage option.
Stuff for the Pantry
The following seasonings can be stored within the pantry the use of an airtight container:
Brown sugar
Chili powder Cinnamon Curry powder Cumin
Italian seasoning
Low-sodium soy sauce Pepper
Salt Vinegar
Olive oil, canola oil, and cooking spray are commonly stocked in the pantry shelf.
Likewise, cooking substances packed in boxes, cans, and jars are stocked inside the
pantry shelves or drawers. Keep the subsequent on hand to your pantry:
Black beans Brown rice Bulgur Chickpeas Diced tomatoes

Dried fruits: apricots, raisins, etc. Dried lentils
Light tuna chunks Oatmeal
Seeds; flaxseed, pumpkin, sunflower Spaghetti sauce
Whole grain pasta
Cooking wines (unopened) along with white and purple wine, balsamic vinegar, etc.

Chapter five How to Eat Out
Fortunately, the Mediterranean food plan isn't always a completely restrictive meal that
eating out while you're on this food regimen might be a big challenge, if no longer
definitely impossible. You can even drink red wine. The important meals restrictions you
are to do not forget when eating out are purple meat, high-fat dairy, and subtle grains.
There are lots of restaurants which give delectable vegetable and seafood dishes in their
menu. With rising technology, you could even surf the internet for restaurants serving
Mediterranean cuisine and examine their menu.
When you consume out, the greatest threat of spoiling any gains you've got finished from
following the MD is exceeding your calories and over-ingesting. Restaurant servings are
historically larger than those we have at home, most particularly if you are the one
making ready your MD. It wouldn't hurt to put together a listing of the maximum amount
of meals items you can still consist of two your dine-out meal. Limit the part of the
servings you consume.

Call the eating place where you plan to dine out and ask questions about how their dishes are prepared. It is your proper to know these items as a consumer. If you're fond of pasta, you may ask if they may be using complete grain pasta. If they don't, you could make a request for a unique meal of entire grain pasta. The sauce want no longer be red meat or red meat given that there are restaurants who serve spaghetti in tuna sauce. You can also request that as opposed to the use of butter or animal fats or oil with Trans fats use extra virgin olive oil.

Special arrangements can continually be made with restaurants especially in case you are a regular. Opt now not to have cheese to your pasta.Dining out means socializing with other people. Make certain to experience consuming your meals with your friends and own family and devour very slowly. As your serving is predicted to be more than the everyday MD serving, you can continually set aside the precise component that you need and feature the waiter percent the rest "to go" before you even start ingesting. Perhaps, if another member of your circle of relatives is likewise on the MD, you can share meals.

a fish dish rather than pink meat, pork or chicken. Select dishes which are not prepared using an excessive amount of oil or butter. The manner of food preparation will serve as clues to the oil/fat content material of the dish. Opt for broiled or grilled dishes, in addition to seared or steamed ones. If your buddies are amenable, you may dine out in Mediterranean restaurants. There should be a pair or extra of such restaurants on your city.

Dining out isn't always in reality a hassle for individuals who followed the Mediterranean eating regimen in their lifestyle. Dining out is not truly a problem for people who followed the Mediterranean weight-reduction plan of their lifestyle.

Chapter 6 Mediterranean Diet: Maintenance Meal Plan
Reality Check
Some people embark on a weight-reduction plan regimen as part of a weight loss goal. This is precisely the objective for penning this eBook. However, each person who desires of dropping weight the usage of the MD or any other diet plan must be in synch with reality. If you won weight over the route of several weeks to a month because of low physical hobby and/or eating extra than your body's energy requirements, you would have packed between five to 7 pounds. This book's -week diet plan in Chapter 3 plus enough exercise and sunshine will really be very powerful for your goal weight aim. While clinical practitioners and other experts do no longer have a single consensus on the secure weight reduction rate, the safest quantity is in the range of one 1/2 to pounds in a week. Therefore, if your aim is to lose 7 pounds in two weeks, that might be pretty safe.

If you've got packed in 30 pounds over the path of to three years, that could be a one of a kind story.

If you move down with the aid of one pound over the path of weeks, you misplaced weight protection and normally. If you misplaced 4 to 6 kilos in weeks, rejoice! You have achieved very well. Yet whether you are within the first or 2d case, you have not lost all the 30 pounds yet inside the aforementioned example. That is what this bankruptcy is for. In fact, even the case cited within the first paragraph desires to go through Chapter 7 - the upkeep plan.

For the cause of the maintenance plan, individuals whose aim is 7 kilos or much less of weight reduction have been performed will be known as Case A, whereas those whose intention is over 7 pounds of weight reduction or those who have not attained their target weight reduction dreams will be called Case B. Separate maintenance plans are drawn for the two cases.

Maintenance Plan: Case A- Target Weight Achieved in 2 Weeks

1. For the ones who have accomplished their goal weight within 2 weeks, the subsequent week (1/3 week) is the transition towards the preservation phase. In the transition phase, one will determine whether or not to place in greater carbs or more variety of carbs in his/her MD (Plan A) or retain with the usual low-carbs intake of the MD for the preceding weeks (Plan S; S for popularity quo or no change).

1. In Plan A, the maintenance plan is to slightly increase carbs intake, either with the aid of increasing the helping a 1/2 of the preceding two weeks however using the equal carbohydrate parts of the 2-week plan or having more leeway. For example, instead of lower-calorie brown rice desserts for the Greek pita recipe, the real pita may be used. One has the loose preference of any of the recipes supplied in Chapter 8.

1. As the time period repute quo suggests, Plan S will preserve the equal low-carbs method as within the previous two weeks. One may pick out any from the recipes in Chapter 8 besides for the Pasta / Bread / Rice category.

1. After the 1/three week, weights are checked again. If folks who used Plan A both continued losing their weight as in the -week plan or maintained their achieved target weight, they may use Plan A as their normal renovation plan.

1. Those who used Plan S and continued dropping their weight as inside the -week plan or maintained their completed target weight can now use Plan A as their preservation plan.

1. Repeat steps 4 or 5 due to the fact the case may be for the fourth week.

1. If folks who chose Plan A or Plan S begin to advantage weight after every week of the plan, revert lower again to the 2-week MD weight reduction plan.

1. After two weeks, look at the equal steps of this preservation plan.

1. It will do no harm if you decide to hold longer with the renovation plan until you experience alarming weight loss rate, which could be very unlikely.

Maintenance Plan: Case B - Target Weight Not Achieved in 2 Weeks

1. For the ones who've not finished their target weight inside 2 weeks, the subsequent week (1/3 week) is the begin of the renovation plan.

1. For simplicity and convenience, one mixes and fits his/her favored menu form the low-carbs MD eating regimen at some stage in the first weeks. The rules are simple:

a. Foods for breakfast from the time table in Chapter 3 may be used for breakfast lunch or dinner, but no longer for snack.

B. The identical rule applies for lunch and dinner elements.

C. Snack ingredients from the schedule in Chapter three may simplest be used as snack.

D. If you need to strive any of the recipes in Chapter 8, please revel in unfastened to do so.

1. After the 1/3 week, weights are checked again. Those who either continued losing their weight as inside the two-week can use Plan A from Case A as their normal maintenance plan. Going over Plan A, the maintenance plan is to slightly increase carbs intake, both via growing the helping a 1/2 of the previous weeks but the use of the equal carbohydrate factors of the -week plan or having greater leeway. For example, as opposed to decrease-calorie brown rice desserts for the Greek pita recipe, the real pita may be used. One has the free desire of any of the recipes provided in Chapter 8.

Chapter 7 Mediterranean Diet: Food for Kids

At this factor to your reading, you'll be questioning if children can even grow wholesome with a Mediterranean weight loss plan. The choice is simpler for other older contributors of the family as it will be handier to prepare the MD weight loss program if all of us or almost everybody is into it. Here are some facts which may help making a decision whether or not or not to educate children in advance for the Mediterranean lifestyle:

One of each 400 kids and adolescents in the US suffers from diabetes.

More than 1 / 4 of Americans less than 20 years of age, which translate to 215,000 young people, have diabetes.

Over one third of children and adolescents in the US are either overweight or overweight; over the past 3 decades, the superiority of youth obesity in the US has doubled; seven in every 10 obese teens develop at the least one danger thing for coronary heart disease.

Obese adolescents tend to broaden to pre-diabetes or high blood sugar levels, which heightens the hazard of diabetes.

Now that the photo is clearer, no one would want their children to maintain with the cutting-edge American kid's weight loss plan of hamburgers, fries, chocolates, and too many sweets. It is by no means early for young youngsters to be brought to the heart-wholesome way of life of the kiddie Mediterranean eating regimen.

Carbohydrates-containing food is most frequently eaten up with the aid of each adults and youngsters. Training kids to consume healthful means teaching them to eat plant starches that are the most essential carbohydrates of the diet. Plant starches are found in the produce phase of grocery shops and supermarkets, especially from fresh culmination and vegetables.

With the surge of weight problems and diabetes costs among youngsters, dad and mom have to educate kids about foods that will affect their glycemic index (GI). This index is a measure of how a lot the blood sugar will increase in a given length after consuming at least 50 grams of carbohydrates. When children devour high GI meals, the pancreas generally tend to produce immoderate amounts of insulin. This, in turn results within the deposition of fats in cells which put kids at hazard for numerous diseases, inclusive of cardiovascular conditions.

Even if carbs and sugar intake among kids need to be controlled, parents cannot maintain their youngsters on low-fat diet because it's far unhealthy to accomplish that and will maximum likely stunt their growth. However, kids need to be exposed to the good fat, fat from plants and from fish and other seafood. Olive oil and other monosaturated fat will help hold the kids' heart healthy and decrease the risk of weight problems and cardiovascular diseases. Moreover, kids' food plans have to contain best protein.

The following tables gift what proteins, carbohydrates and fats need to be fed on by using children in the Mediterranean weight-reduction plan and people which need to not be eaten.

List of carbohydrates which ought to be eaten by children the ones which they need to avoid.

CONSUME or EMPHASIZE THESE sensible FATS AVOID or LIMIT CONSUMPTION of those UNHEALTHY FATS

Almonds Butter

Cashew round the bend Fats from meat

Fish oils (DHA and EPA) Fatty meats

Macadamia round the bend Fats from cooked foods

Peanuts

Unprocessed spread

Walnuts

Table 3: List of proteins that should be enclosed in children's diet those which they ought to avoid.

CONSUME or EMPHASIZE THESE PROTEINS AVOID or LIMIT CONSUMPTION of those UNHEALTHY PROTEINS

Broiled or baked fish Fatty beef cuts and hamburger

Eggs meat and lunch meats

Lean beef cooked super molecule foods

Milk proteins: whey and casein

Skim milk

Skinless chicken, turkey breast

Soy

Table four illustrates the ingredients that have low, mild, and excessive glycemic index. kids required to be right educated around foods and their corresponding class primarily based entirely on glycemic index in order that they will preserve on with the Mediterranean weight loss program even after they are at school. Packing snacks for the youngsters can diminish the possibility of buying unhealthy food after they is also not beneath the watchful eyes of their oldsters.

Table four. samples of ingredients with low, slight and excessive GI.

CONSUME or EMPHASIZE CONSUME MODERATELY LIMIT or AVOID CONSUMPTION

Low GI Moderate GI High GI

(GI below fifty) (GI from 50 to 75) (GI over 75)

Apple Balance Bar Cakes

Butter Banana Carrots

Fructose rice Cookies

Grapes Corn Cornflakes
Lentils Mixed-grain breads aldohexose
Low-carb bars Oatmeal High-carb bars
Meat (lean) Potato chips Potatoes
Milk Table sugar Pretzels
Navy beans Sweet potatoes Raisins
Peanuts preserved nuts
Pinto beans chopped wheat
Protein-enriched food breadstuff
Soy rice
Healthy kids are happy children. Guide them through the Mediterranean diet currently. it's ne'er too early to worry for his or her health.

Chapter eight Recipes for Mediterranean Weight Loss Diet
Here are the foremost luxurious weight reduction recipes of the Mediterranean diet. They style therefore scrumptious properly you won't even note your wanting to shed off pounds. attempt them for your room with the bonus bankruptcy on recommendations for a success Mediterranean preparation. for each formula, a code within the form 4S/BLD, that shows:
S simply prior the slash suggests servings and therefore the vary earlier than S is that the style of servings.
BLD when the slash suggests breakfast, lunch, or dinner. If S is visible when the slash, it indicates that the food is also consumed as dish

Fish
Salmon-Asparagus dish (Frittata) 4S /BLD
Sumptuous however wholesome salmon and asparagus dish sauté
 the standard Mediterranean method.
Ingredients:
Quantity live Food Item
2 tbsp. (10 ml.) Dried dill
1 cup (250 millilitre.) ingredient or egg substitute
0.25 tbsp. (1.25 ml.) Ground black pepper
2 tbsp. (30 ml.) additional virgin oil
0.25 cup (60 millilitre.) Feta cheese (crumbled fine)
0.25 tbsp. (1.25 ml.) ocean salt or kosher salt to style (Note: is also lessened particularly if the salmon is salty or as preferred)
0.25 pound (115 g.) Sliced salmon (smoked)
1 pound (450 g.) Stalks of asparagus cut in one in. or 2.5 cm. pieces
0.5 tbsp. (2.5 ml.) Tarragon
Directions:
1. place asparagus and oil in a very medium length ovenproof cooking pan and heat for three minutes or till the stalks soften. Add dill, pepper, salt and tarragon. Stir gently for a second.

1. place within the eggs within the higher than combination followed now via the salmon and feta cheese that need to be frivolously distributed. Cook till the eggs are firm while not overlaying the cooking pan.

1. take away from heat and region cooking pan at the kitchen appliance rack around half-dozen inches underneath the broiler. Broil the weather from three to five minutes or until high of the egg turns brown.

1. take away from broiler and serve. Baked Salmon with Honey-Balsamic Glaze

Quantity

4 Measure

tbsp. (60 ml.) Food Item

Balsamic vinegar

1 tbsp. (15 ml.) metropolis mustard

3 cloves Garlic (minced)

1 tbsp. (15 ml.) Honey

2 tbsp. Oregano (fresh, chopped)

0.25 tbsp. (1.25 ml.) Ground black pepper

4 four ounces Salmon filets

0.25 tbsp. (1.25 ml.) Salt to style

1 tbsp. (15 ml.) wine

4S/BLD (Note: Salmon may be replaced with halibut)

Ingredients:

Directions:

1. Routine baking preparation manner: Line baking sheet with aluminum foil; spray with canola oil cooking spray (usually PAM cooking spray); preheat oven to 400 °F.

1. Put salt and pepper on salmon filets.

1. Glaze preparation manner:

a. Coat a small sauce pan with cooking spray or a little canola oil.

B. Sauté garlic in medium heat for three minutes or until it is soft.

C. Mix honey, mustard, salt, vinegar and wine. Add to the cooked garlic.

D. Simmer without cowl in medium or low warmness for 3 minutes or until the glaze barely thickens.

E. Remove from warmness and set aside half of the glaze in every other container.

1. Baking procedure for the salmon:

a. Arrange the salmon at the baking sheet with the pores and skin-facet down.

B. Brush every piece of salmon with the last glaze within the saucepan.

C. Sprinkle the glazed salmon with oregano on top.

D. Bake for about 10 minutes or until salmon flakes effortlessly with a fork.

E. Transfer the fish to plates the usage of a turner, but depart the skin on the foil.

F. Brush the baked salmon with the glaze set aside in advance Sesame Tuna Temptation 6S/BLD (Note: Traditionally, this recipe is known as Tuna Carpaccio, an appetizer, but in a weight loss plan, this is already a complete meal when a cup or less of culmination in season is fed on after this course. For decrease carbohydrate content, simple rice cakes organized from brown rice was substituted for the pita bread.)

Directions:

1. Mix ginger, garlic, sesame oil and seeds, and soy well. Encrust the tuna in the mixture.
1. Heat a sauté pan to the very best degree and pan-sear the tuna.
1. Add the seared tuna and the scallions to the sauce mixture.
1. Garnish with quartered apple.
1. Eat the dish with the obvious rice cakes

Dessert

Apple-Walnut Delight 6S/BLDS

Ingredients:

Quantity Measure Food Item

4 pieces Apples (medium, Rome or Gala variety, and diced into ¼ inch cubes

eight pieces Apricots (dried)

2 tbsp. Honey

1 tbsp. Olive oil

½ piece Orange (use juice and zest)

½ cup Walnuts (toasted and chopped

Directions:

1. Whisk the orange juice and zest, together with honey and olive oil in a salad serving bowl.
1. Add the apples and apricots. Toss those 2 fruits to coat then with the aggregate in Step 1.
1. Add the chopped walnuts, toss and serve. Fruit Salad Mediterranean Style

6S/BLDS

Ingredients:

Quantity Measure Food Item

½ Cup Almonds (toasted and chopped)

4 Pieces Fuyu persimmons (sliced into 10 wedges)

1 ½ Cups Grapes (reduce into halves)

1 tbsp. Honey

1 tbsp. Lemon Juice

8 Pieces Mints leaves (rolled and sliced thinly)

Directions:

1. Combine all the components in a salad serving bowl.
1. Toss and serve.

Legumes

Chickpea and Barley Glee 6S/BLDS

Ingredients:

Quantity Measure Food Item

1 cup Apricots (diced, dried)

¼ tsp. Cardamom

1 cup Chicken broth or as an alternative, vegetable broth

½ tsp. Cinnamon

½ tsp. Ginger

1 dash Hot sauce

2 portions Lemon (juice and zest)

¼ cup Olive oil

1 cup Parsley (discard the stems and chop finely)

½ cup Pearl barley

¼ tsp. Pepper

1 cup Pistachio nuts (shelled)

1 piece Red onion (thinly sliced)

pinch Salt to taste

8 cups Spinach (toddler spinach) leaves

¼ tsp. Turmeric

Directions:

Put the broth in a small sauce pan. Bring the broth to a boil using excessive warmth. Add the pearl barley and cover.

Remove the pan from the warmth and set aside for 15 minutes.

1. Combine the apricots, chickpeas, lemon juice and zest, olive oil. Parsley, purple onion, and the spices in a blending bowl. Put in the warm sauce and salt to taste.

2. Garnish by using arranging the infant spinach leaves on a serving platter. Add the chickpeas and barley aggregate on top of the leaves.

1. Top the salad meal with pistachios and serve.

Meat Lamb Loin Chops 4S/LD

Ingredients:

Quantity Measure Food Item

½ cup couscous (organized from whole wheat grains)

1 piece Cucumber (medium, peeled, chopped)

2 tbsp. Dill (fresh and finely chopped)

½ cup Feta cheese (crumbled)

1 tbsp. Garlic (minced)

2 pounds (or 8 pcs) Lemon juice

1 tbsp. Parsley (fresh and finely chopped)

2 tbsp. Olive oil (extra virgin)

¼ tsp. Salt

2 pieces Tomatoes (medium, chopped)

1 cup Water

Directions:

1. Boil water in a medium-length sauce pan.

1. To prepare the couscous:

a. Stir inside the couscous into the boiling water from Step 1.

B. Bring to a boil and reduce warmness just to simmer, cowl the pan, and wait for 5 minutes.

C. Use fork to fluff the simmering couscous-water mix.

D. Transfer to combination to a container.

E. Add the cucumber, dill, feta, lemon juice, and tomatoes to the couscous, and stir. Pour the couscous aggregate into the lamb loin chops and serve.

1. To put together the lamb loin chops:

a. Mix the minced garlic, parsley and salt in a bowl. Put the mixture into the chops by using pressing it onto the loin.

B. Heat olive oil into a non-stick pan or skilled using from medium to high warmth level. Put the lamb loin chops into the hot oil till it is cooked.

This will take approximately 10 to twelve minutes.

C. Set aside however preserve warm.

Ground Round Special a Los Angeles Turk

4S/LD

Ingredients:

Quantity Measure Food Item

1/8 tsp. Allspice (ground)

1/three cup Breadcrumbs (dry)

1/four tsp. Cinnamon (ground)

Cooking spray

Half of tsp. Cumin (ground)

1 piece Egg (huge, overwhelmed lightly)

1 tsp. Garlic (used bottled, minced)

1 pound Ground round sirloin or any lean pork cut

1/four cup Mint (fresh, chopped)

Half cup Onion (white, chopped)

Four portions (6 inches) Pita bread (split)

2 portions Plum tomatoes (sliced, four to six slices per piece)

1/four tsp. Red pepper (ground)

Half tsp. Salt

1 tbsp. Tomato paste

1/four cup Yogurt (low-fat, plain)

Directions:

1. Preheat the broiler in instruction for cooking.

1. Mix the subsequent components in a bowl: allspice, breadcrumbs, cinnamon, cumin, egg, garlic, ground round red meat, mint, onion, pink pepper, salt, and tomato paste.

 Stir till the components combine well.

1. Prepare 8 to 12 pieces of patty from the mixture in Step 2.

1. Put cooking spray in a jelly roll pan and place the patties within the oil-coated pan.

1. Broil each sides of the patty for a total of 10 to 15 minutes relying on your choice of how executed the patties are.

1. Fill in each half of the pita bread with a patty and a slice of tomato.

1. Garnish every patty-crammed pita with yogurt.

.

Relish the goodness of Mediterranean meat cuisine in this ground spherical special Relish the goodness of Mediterranean meat cuisine on this ground spherical special

Pasta / Rice / Bread

Breakfast Rush

5-7S/BS (Note: When this dish is consumed for snack, the meal plan in Chapter 3 calls it Snack Pack) Ingredients:

Quantity Measure Food Item

1 cup Banana (sliced)

1 cup Granola

1 cup Multigrain cereals

½ cup Raisins

1 cup Rolled oats

1 cup Other fresh or frozen fruit as preferred

½ cup Walnuts or almonds

1 cup Whole grain cereals

2 cup Almond, skim, or soy milk (low-fat)

1 cup Yogurt (plain, low fat or fats-free) Directions:

1. In a massive salad bowl or container (with volume at the least 12 cups or three liters or 1 gallon,

Integrate the cereals and the oats. If there may be no container massive enough, divide the ingredients into identical batches of 4.

1. Add the nits and culmination and mix well, but gently.

1. Add within the milk and the yogurt.

1. Pack in smaller packing containers with cover and keep in freezer for no more than 2 days. Brown Rice Pudding

6S/BS (Note: When this dish is consumed for snack, the meal plan in Chapter three calls it Snack Pack) Ingredients:

Quantity Measure Food Item

½ cup Almonds

½ cup Brown rice

½ cup Butter (low-fat or light)

½ tsp. Cardamom

Four cups Milk

1 tbsp. Orange (zest only)

¼ cup Raisins

½ tsp. Rose water (might not be used if preferred)

Directions:

1. Soak the rice for 10 to 15 minutes in water. Drain

1. Boil the milk and sugar in a sauce pan in medium or excessive warmth to a low boil.

Add the cardamom, cinnamon, raisins, and drained rice & convey the mix to a simmer over low warmness.

 Wait for the mixture to thicken earlier than disposing of from warmness. This takes about forty five minutes of simmering with common stirring required.

2. Remove from the burner, upload the rose water (whilst preferred).

1. Prepare the almonds and the zest of orange mixture.

1. Use a ladle to transfer the pudding from the pan to serving bowls and top with the almond and orange zest aggregate.

1. May be served hot or chilled.

Walnut Baklava

32S/BS

Ingredients:

Quantity live Food Item

½ cup Butter (low-fat or lightweight, melted)

1 tbsp. Cardamom

2 tbsp. Cinnamon

2 items Cinnamon (sticks)

½ cup Honey

1 tbsp. juice

1 tsp. Lemon (zest)

½ cup oil

2 tsp. Orange (zest)

½ pound puff paste dough (approximately twenty sheets)

¼ and 1½ cups Sugar

three cups Walnuts

1 ½ cup Water

2 cups Pistachios

Directions:

1. Routine baking practice procedure: heat kitchen appliance to 325 °F.

1. place cinnamon sticks, honey, juice, 1½ cups sugar, and water in an exceedingly serious sauce pan. boil medium to excessive hotness for twenty minutes.

take away pan from hotness, put aside and funky at intervals the electric refrigerator, however remove the cinnamon sticks initial.

1. place the cardamom, cinnamon, the ultimate sugar and zests in an exceedingly meals processor and set to route chop (30 pulses).

1. combine butter and oil and brush the mixture on the edges of the baking pan victimization storage room brush.

1. Unroll the puff paste and cut back in halves.

1. place one sheet at the pan, brush with butter-oil mixture and repeat the procedure until all sheets had been brushed.

1. Bake for one hours and pour the honey. put aside for thirty minutes before serving.

Poultry

Brown Rice and Stuffed Chicken

10S/LD (Note: unremarkably served throughout lunch or dinner, however it's your meal. no one can forestall you if you would like to own it for breakfast.)

Ingredients:

Quantity live Food Item

2 cups stock

1 piece Chicken (whole, weighs or so five pounds, suspend giblets)

1 piece Lemon (zest)

¼ cup Olives (green)

2 tbsp. And the other one tbsp. Olive oil

1 piece Onion (medium sized; chopped)

1 tsp. Paprika

1 tsp. Pepper

½ cup Pine balmy

1 cup rice

½ teaspoon Salt

2 cups wine (dry)

Directions:

1. heat the kitchen appliance set to 350 °F.

1. Toss the pine balmy in medium hotness for one minute the employment of a 2-quart sauce pan.

Add the onions and cook by victimization frequent stirring for three minutes.

1. Add the stock and scrape very cheap of the pan to form certain that no balmy stuck.

1. Boil the mix in medium to excessive heat. place the olives and rice, cowl the pan and cut back the warmth while cooking for roughly forty minutes

or until the liquid combination has been absorbed with the help of the rice.

1. place the chook within the roast rack of the open. Rub the inner cavity of the bird with two tbsp. Of oil.

combine within the lemon peel, paprika, pepper, and salt. Rub the spice combination on the fowl. Brush the chook with the final word oil.

2. Stuff the chook with the overdone rice and pour the wine on the surface a part of the chook.

1. Bake the bird while not cowl till the rice and therefore the hen attain AN inner temperature of 1 hundred sixty 5 degrees.

Check internal temperature AN hour once baking.

1. Baste the bird every twenty minutes. The baking time is spherical one ½ hours on the typical.

1. Set apart the fowl to cool down before cutting. take away the rice from the bird hole and transfer into a serving platter.

1. Ideal serving share is two to a couple of oz. of fowl to 1/2 cup of rice.

Salad
Greek Salad 4S/BLD
Ingredients:
Quantity Measure Food Item
2 portions Cucumbers (medium-sized; seeded, diced)
four ounces Feta cheese (crumbled)
1 clove Garlic (minced)
1 piece Lemon (huge, juiced)
½ cup Olives (kalamata variety; pitted, chopped)
1/3 cup Olive oil
¼ cup Parsley (fresh, flat leaves, chopped)
Pepper (to taste)
8 cups Romaine lettuce (torn into chunk size pieces)
Salt (to taste)
4 pieces Tomato (medium sized)
Directions:
1. Put the lettuce in a huge salad bowl
1. Cut the tomatoes into eight wedges every. Place them on top of the lettuce. Add the cucumbers, olives, onions, and parsley.
1. Whisk the following components in a smaller bowl: garlic, lemon juice, and olive oil. Put salt and pepper at the dressing to taste.

Pour this within the mixed greens from Step 1.
1. Sprinkle with feta cheese and serve soon.

Snack
1 or greater S/BS or dessert for a prime meal Frutti Smoothies Galore!
Here are substances for a host of Frutti Smoothie snacks which you can put together in advance to chill inside the freezer.
You may additionally choose to put together the snack a few minutes earlier than you devour your snack,
however for greater fun snacking, the ingredients berries, fruit and liquids ought to be pre-refrigerated.
You can prepare a snack of one serving for yourself or multiple servings for your family. Even youngsters love the smoothies!
Ingredients:
Berries and Fruits Liquids Additional Ingredients
Apple sauce Almond milk Almond butter
Blackberries Apple juice Granola topping
Blueberries Ice Peanut butter
Mango Orange juice Rolled oats
Peaches Skim milk Shredded coconut

Pears Soy milk Soy protein powder

Pineapples Yogurt (low-fats or non-fat) Whey protein powder

Raspberries

Ripe bananas

Strawberries

Combine your desired ingredients in a quantity that will no longer make the use of the blender a challenge.

You may get one or more elements from each category, but use your imagination to concoct super snack and breakfast ideas.

1. Blend them until smooth. You may also add more ice or liquid as needed.

Some smoothie concoctions are shown subsequent page: Frutti Smoothie No. 1

Ripe banana Almond milk Rolled oats Almond butter Ice

Fruity Smoothie No. 2 Pineapples

Orange juice Granola topping Ice

Fruity Smoothie No. three Strawberries Peaches

Skim milk Shredded coconut Ice

Fruity Smoothie No. 4 Apple sauce

Apple Juice Yogurt Rolled oats Ice

Fruity Smoothie No. 5 Blackberries Blueberries

Almond milk Yogurt

Whey protein powder Ice

Just keep blending and matching! Here's Frutti Smoothie No. three. Yummy!

Soup

Carrot Soup

4S/LD (Note: Normally served for the duration of lunch or dinner, but it's your meal. Nobody will prevent you if you need to have it for breakfast.)

Ingredients:

Quantity Measure Food Item

½ cup Apple juice (ideally organic)

2 kilos Carrots (ideally organic; peeled and chopped) 1 or 2 pinch Curry powder or cumin (higher if slight and must be gluten-free)

1 or 2 sprint Sea salt (to taste, better low sodium for health) Water (sparkling and cool)

Directions:

1. Put the chopped carrots in a soup pan (pot) and pour enough water to cowl the carrots by means of approximately an inch.

1. Put a sprint of salt and a few curry powder or cumin. The amount of curry or cumin depends on you

(or your education to the character preparing the meal, but generally a pinch or two is sufficient).

Cover the pan (pot) and boil the carrots. After boiling, lower the heat of the burner and allow simmering until the carrots are gentle to your preferred softness.

 This need to take much less than 30 mins.

 Add greater water if vital if the initial amount of water is not sufficient.

1. Turn the soup right into a puree the usage of a blender. Stop blending as soon because the carrots are combined and the mixture is smooth.

1. Add the apple juice.

1. A version to the menu for the ones who would really like to experiment on a creamy one may be made by means of adding a creamy component
 such as light coconut milk or the unsweetened sort of almond milk instead of apple juice.
Other canned cream products can be used depending to your familiarity with the product.
Lentil Soup (Fakkes)
4S/LD (Note: Normally served at some stage in lunch or dinner, but it's your meal. Nobody will prevent you if you need to have it for breakfast.)
Ingredients:
Quantity Measure Food Item
2 portions Bay leaves
1 piece Carrot (medium sized; chopped finely)
Four cloves Garlic (whole)
1 pound Lentils (dry; this is approximately 2 cups in volume)
½ cup Olive oil (more virgin)
1 piece Onion (medium sized; peeled and grated)
1 teaspoon Rosemary (dried)
1 cup Tomatoes (fresh or canned; minced and sieved)

Water
Directions:
1. Soak the lentils in water overnight.
1. Boil water on a huge pot. Rinse the lentils and put them in boiling water for 10 minutes.
1. Drain the water and placed in another 6 pints of water and boil.
1. As the aggregate boils, add the relaxation of the elements and continue boiling till the lentils are cooked and smooth.

 This commonly takes an hour.
1. Remove the bay leaves and serve.

Vegetables
Eggplant and Tomato Pesto
4S/LD (Note: Normally served at some point of lunch or dinner, however it's your meal. Nobody will forestall you ,if you need to have it for breakfast.)
Ingredients:
Quantity Measure Food Item
1 cup Basil leaves (upload approximately 15 greater leaves for stacking)
Cooking spray (non-stick)
1 piece Eggplant (sliced spherical, ½ inch)
1 cup Feta cheese (crumbled)
1 clove Garlic
1 piece Lemon (zest and juice)
2 tbsp. Pine nuts
2 tbsp. Olive oil
Pepper (to taste)
2 to three portions Rome tomatoes or beefsteak tomatoes (sliced round, ½ inch)
Salt (to taste)
1 ½ tsp. Sea salt

Directions:

Extract bitterness from the eggplant by means of rubbing them with salt and topping them with salt afterwards. Set apart for 30 minutes.

Rinse afterwards and pat them dry.

1. Blend 1 cup of basil leaves, garlic, lemon juice and zest, olive oil, pine nits, salt, and paper in a blender for 2 to a few mins or till the pesto smoothens. Set aside.

1. Spray the eggplant very gently with the cooking spray. The grill ought to additionally be sprayed on.

1. Heat the grill to medium or excessive heat. Grill both sides of each eggplant round from 3 to 5 minutes or till the favored texture is achieved.

2. Each serving encompass one eggplant round, 1 tsp. Of pesto, 1 slices of tomato, and a basil leaf. Top all of the garnished eggplants with crumbled feta.

Serve.

Bonus - high Seven Tips for flourishing Mediterranean preparation

Tip No. 1:

Nuts and/or could also be wet on breakfast cereal or ready as home-brewed spreads, significantly peanuts or spread. However, if you're exploitation merchandise from the food market, browse the label to form positive that the sugar and fat content, particularly if you're getting ready MD recipes for weight loss.

Nuts/seeds can also be wet to dairy product for snacks. Tip No. 2:

Other nice uses for nutty and seeds within the room are:

Chopped nutty or seeds are nice for bread toppings once baking; Use nuts and seeds for crunchier salads or alimentary paste dishes; Toast benny seeds and add these to your stir-fries exploitation healthy nut oils.

Tip No. 3:

Nuts are associate degree everyday staple within the Mediterranean diet as they're utilized in desserts, salads, and a few aspect dishes.

Use glass and plastic containers that are airtight; Store nutty off from foods with sturdy odor like garlic as nuts Teddy boy to soak up odor from their surroundings;

Shelled nutty could also be unbroken at temperature for as long as three months and up to four months once refrigerated; Unshelled nutty could last for four months once cold and doubly as long when unbroken within the freezer; If obtainable however nutty from farmers.

Otherwise opt to obtain nutty from stores that you simply have discovered to own a high employee turnover to make sure freshness; It is a lot of well to shop for nutty preplaced with a best before or date to own a thought however long the nuts are up available.

Tip No. 4:

The Mediterranean diet is grounded on the balance of the proper foods as mirrored within the MD pyramid in Chapter eight. to form the pyramid work for you, take into account the subsequent within the preparation of the MD diet

Tip No. 5

Fruits and vegetables: select by season to make sure freshness specialize in wholes: Whole grain, whole fruits and vegetables Fish and shellfish:

Best doubly per week Red meat: little serving once per week Dairy: select solely low-fat or fat free and ensure they extremely are Alcohol:

forever consume in moderate quantity. Herbs and spices are a vicinity of Mediterranean preparation. the subsequent herbs are unremarkably cultivated within

the region: basil, deal, fennel, mint, oregano, parsley, rosemary, sage, and thyme. be happy to incorporate these in your dishes for that ancient

Mediterranean flavor.

Tip No. 6:

Depending on your family's preference, you'll be able to tailor your preparation for specific Mediterranean regions.
Southern Italian preparation uses anchovies, balsams vinegar, basil, bay leaf, capers, garlic, oregano, parsley,
 peppers, among different herbs & spices. To flavor of the Southern Italian Mediterranean preparation is, so zesty with a saucy and spicy hot flavor

Tip No. 7:
Grecian Mediterranean preparation has basil, cucumber, dill, fennel, garlic, honey, lemon, mint, olives (of course), oregano, and yogurt.
Their flavors so run a scale from lemon like with citrus accent to savory and daring or soft flavors with creamy texture

www.ingramcontent.com/pod-product-compliance
Lightning Source LLC
Chambersburg PA
CBHW081922120726
47996CB00010B/3433